Helping Our World Get Well
COVID VACCINES

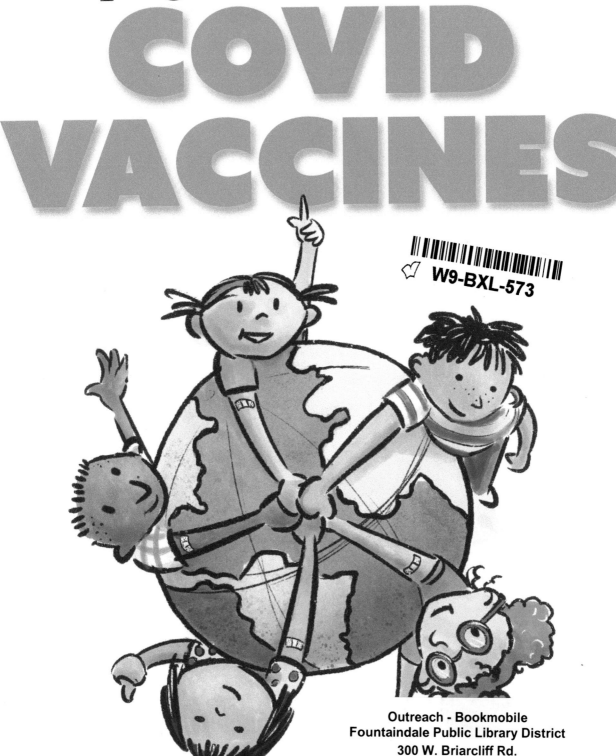

written by Beth Bacon   illustrated by Kary Lee

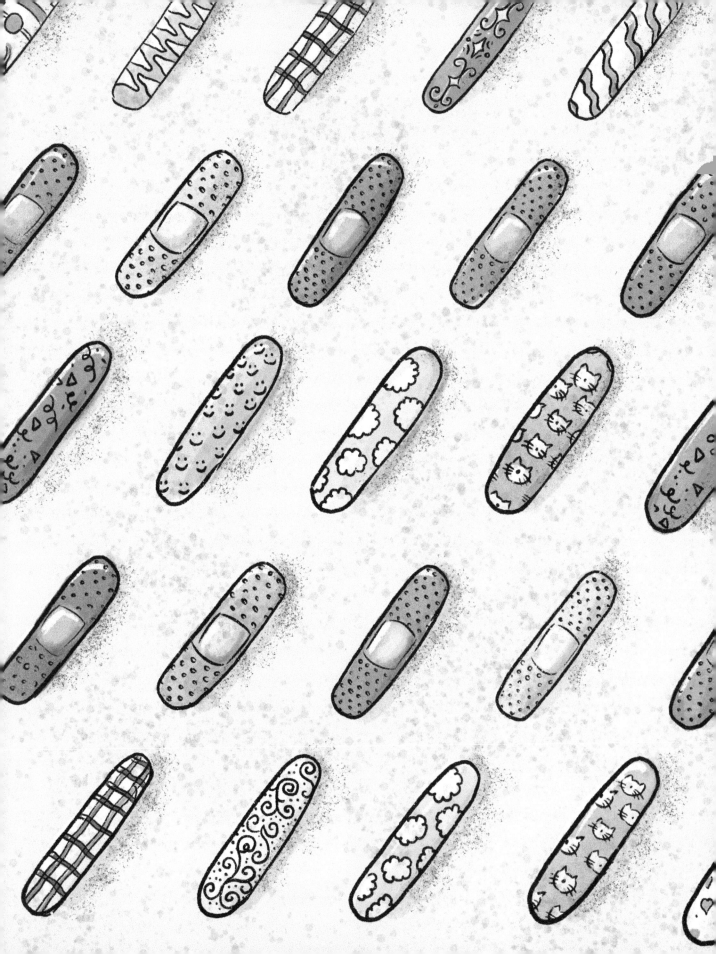

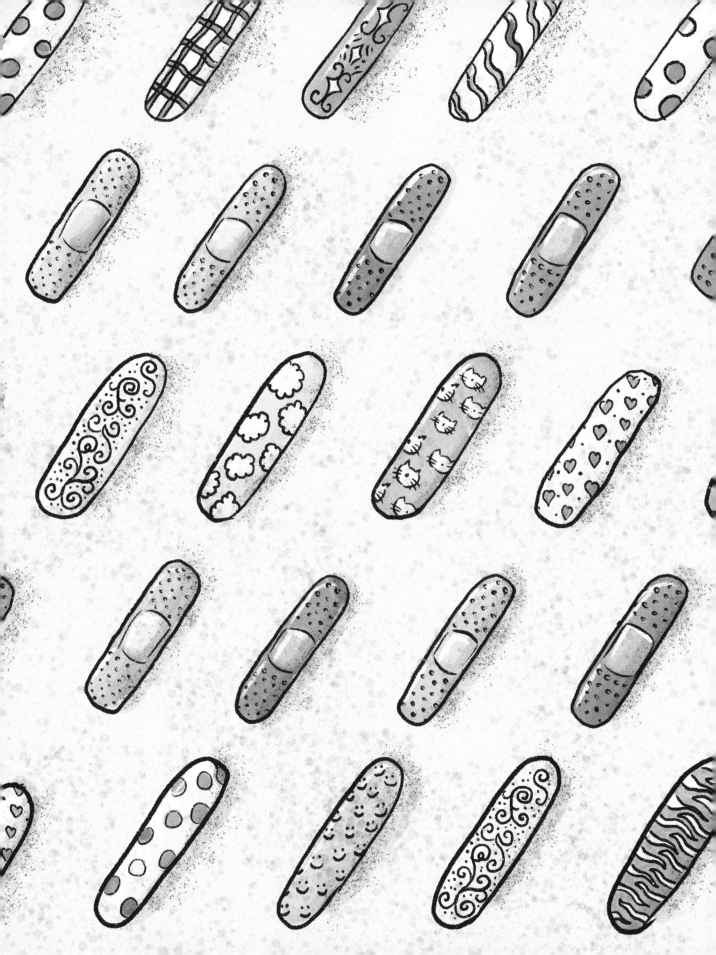

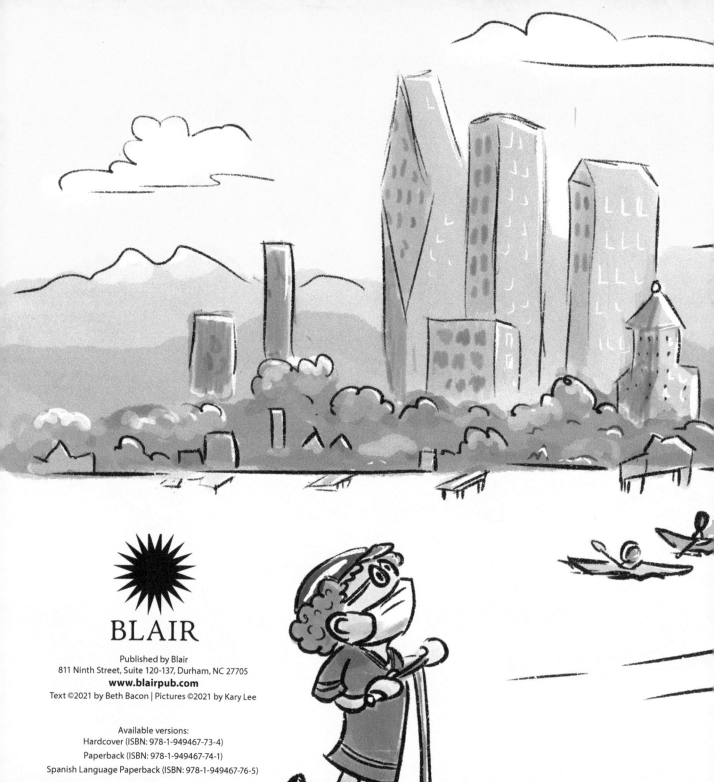

BLAIR

Published by Blair
811 Ninth Street, Suite 120-137, Durham, NC 27705
www.blairpub.com
Text ©2021 by Beth Bacon | Pictures ©2021 by Kary Lee

Available versions:
Hardcover (ISBN: 978-1-949467-73-4)
Paperback (ISBN: 978-1-949467-74-1)
Spanish Language Paperback (ISBN: 978-1-949467-76-5)

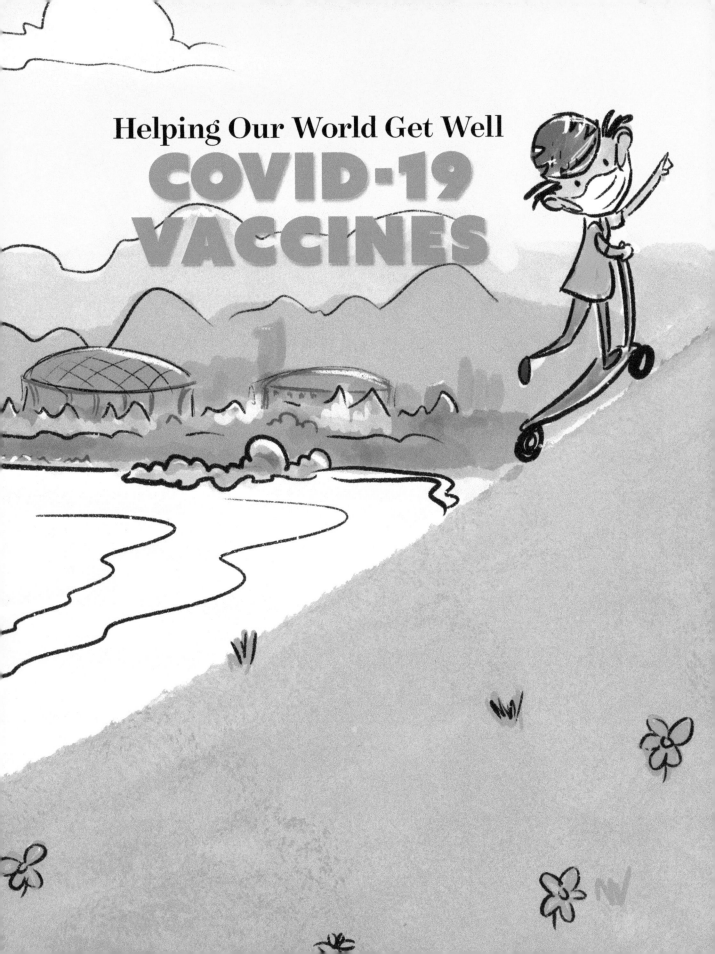

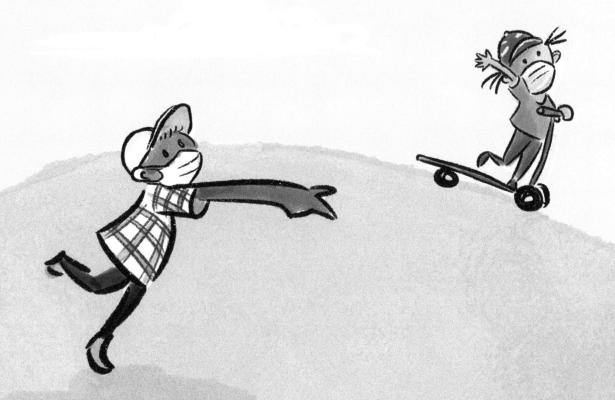

When the coronavirus came to the world,
people did lots of new things to stay healthy.

I wore a mask and we all stayed six feet apart.

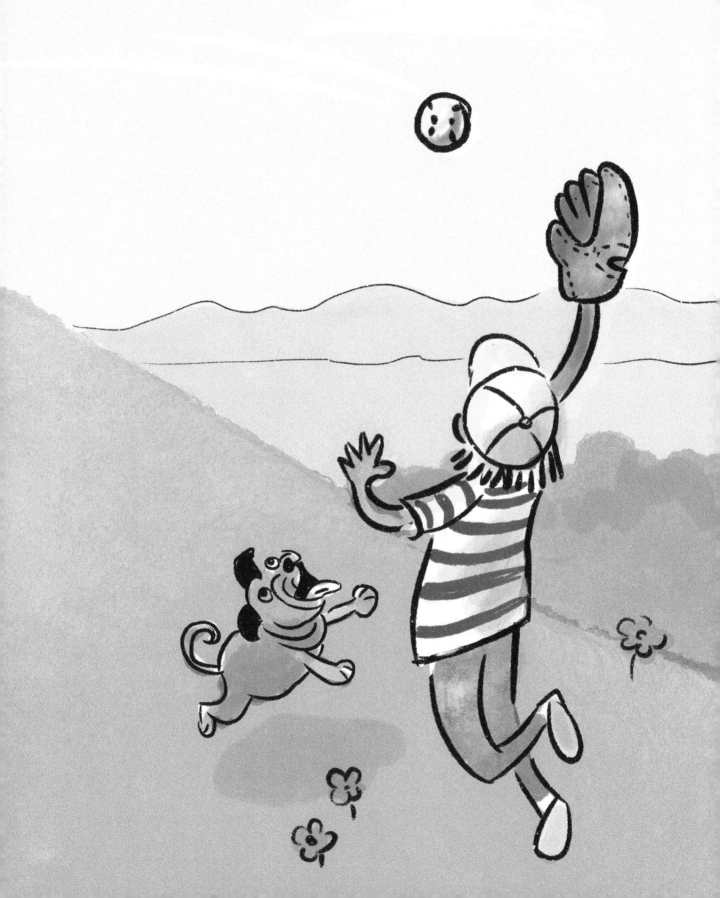

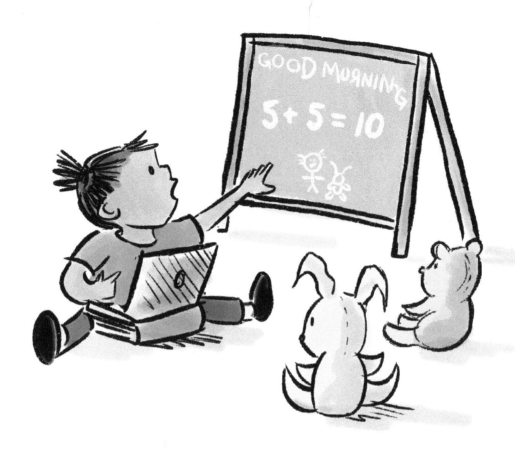

I went to school online and practiced karate outside.

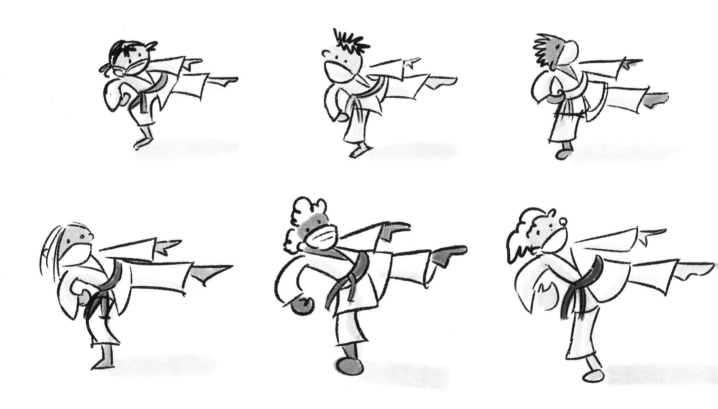

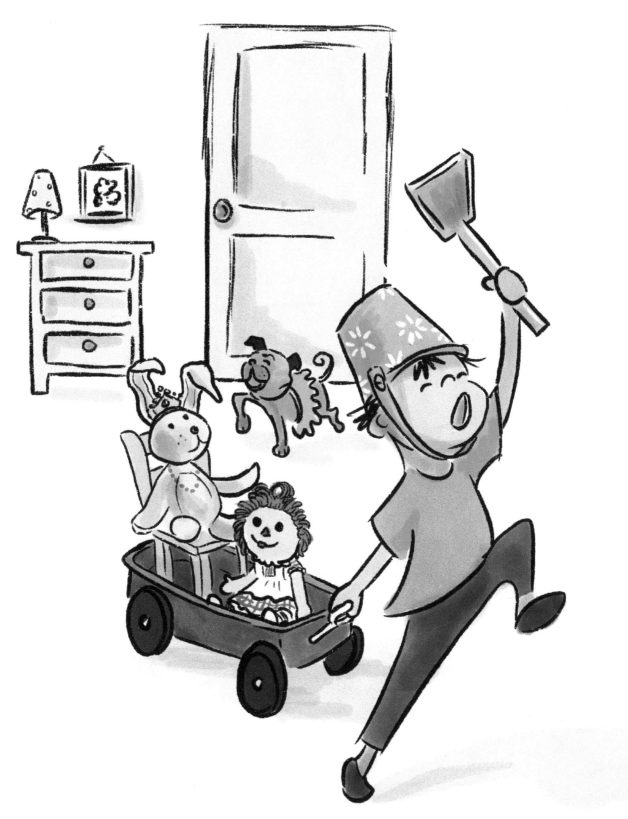

When our summer parade was cancelled,
I started one of my own.

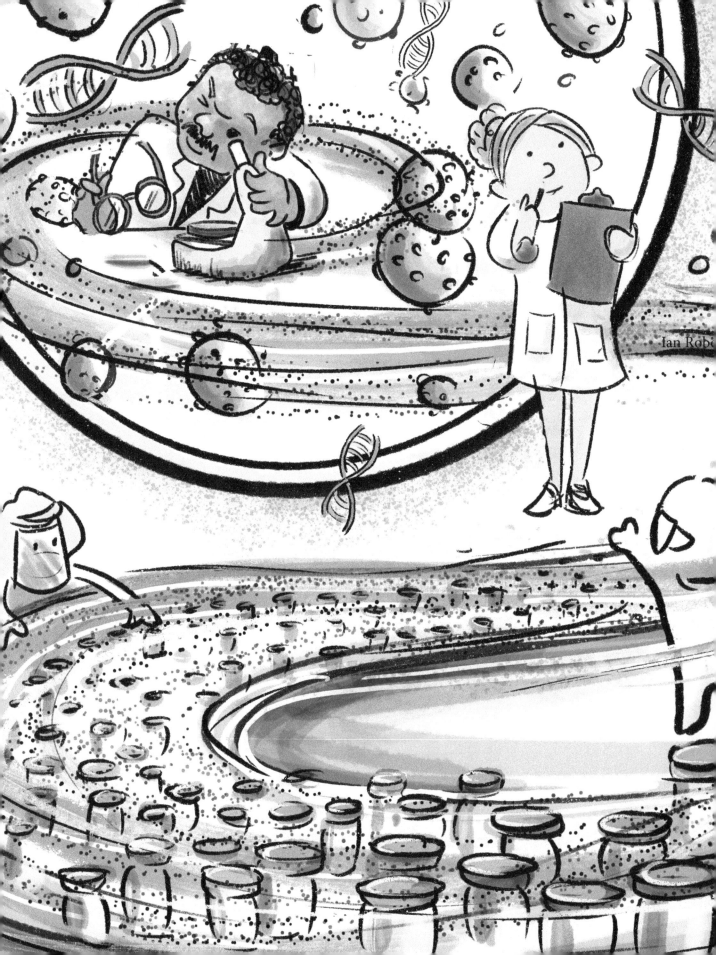

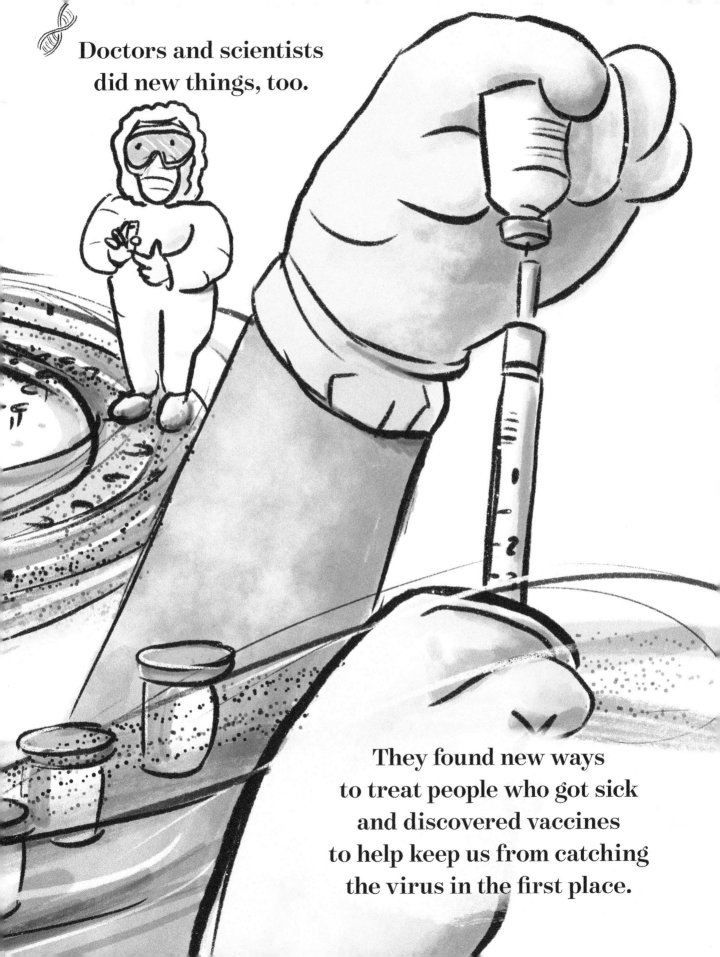

Doctors and scientists did new things, too.

They found new ways to treat people who got sick and discovered vaccines to help keep us from catching the virus in the first place.

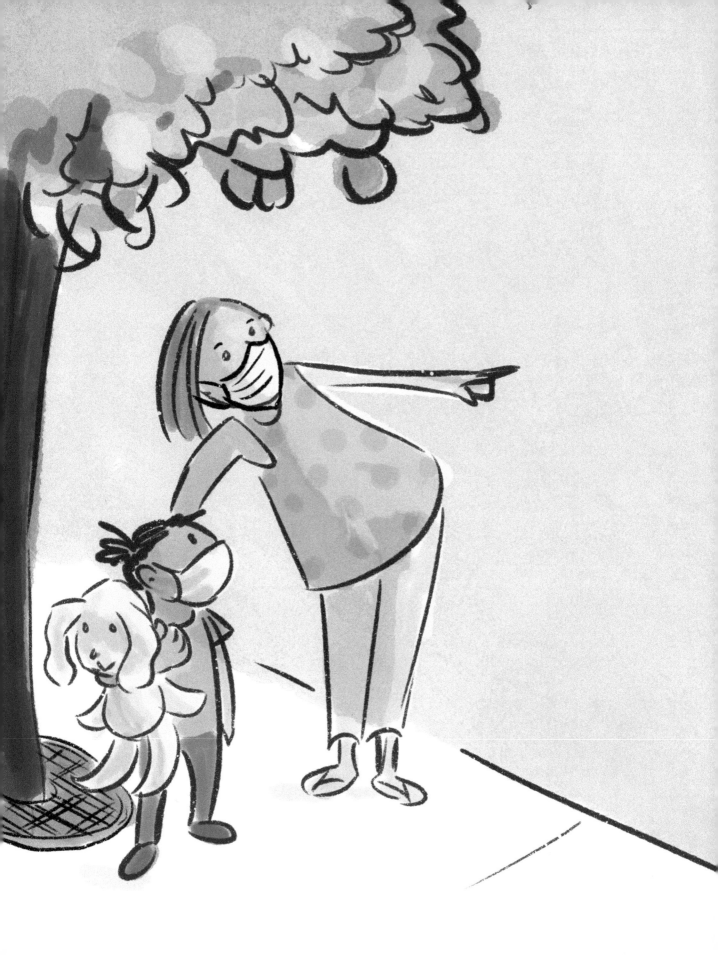

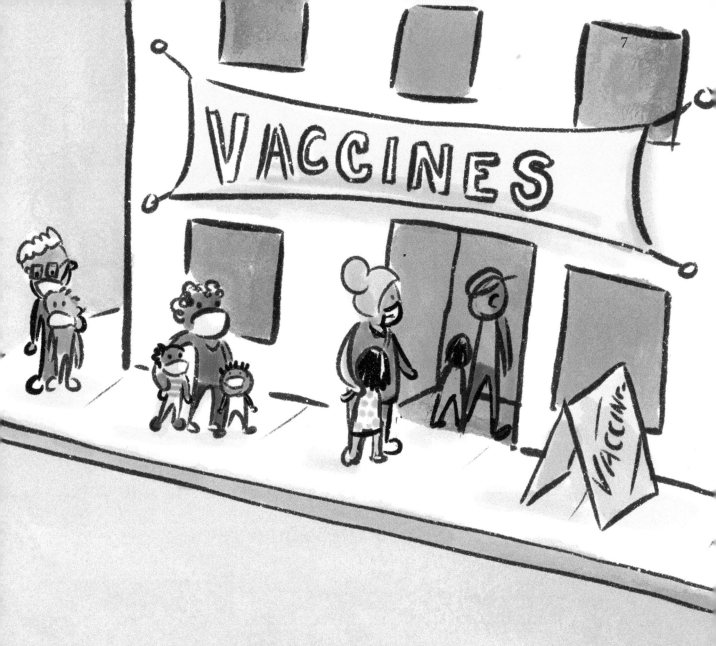

But a Covid vaccine was
one new thing I didn't want
to do. What if it made me cry?
What if it made me bleed?
What if it made me sick?

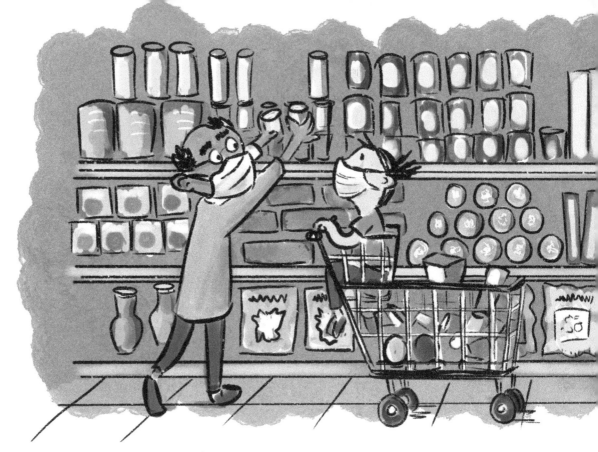

"I got a Covid vaccine," said Grampa Dan.
"Now I worry less when I go to the market."

He made a good point.

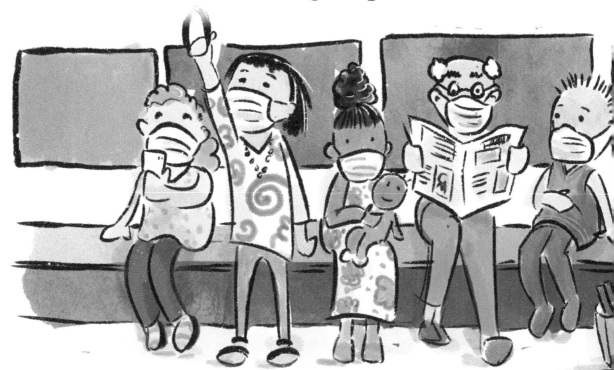

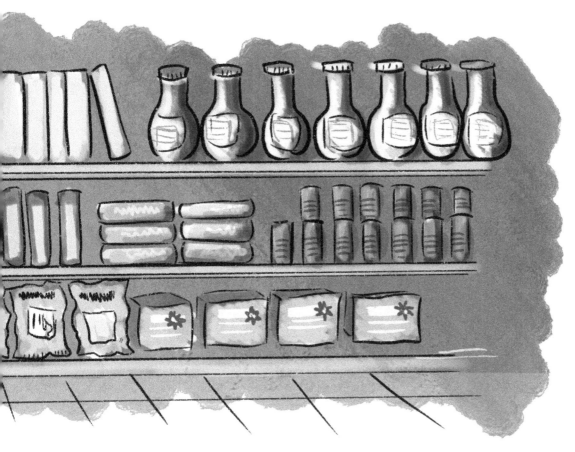

"I had my Covid vaccine," said Tía Rosa.
"Now I feel safer on my way to work."

She made a good point, too.

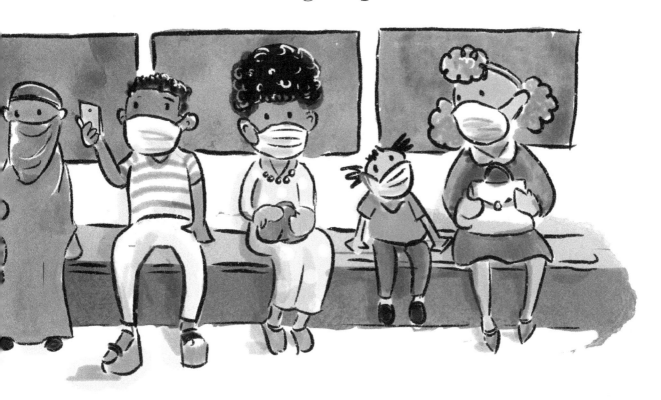

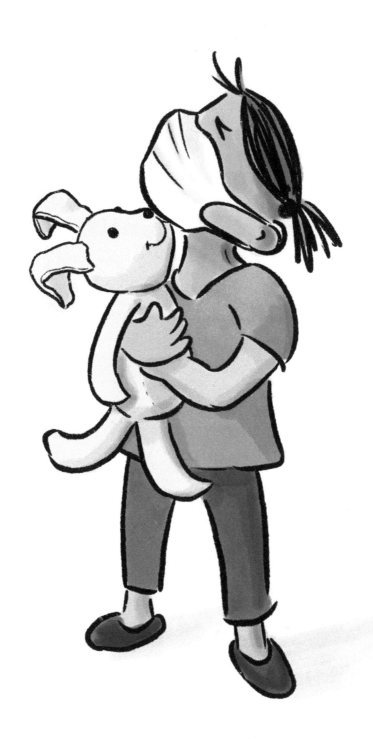

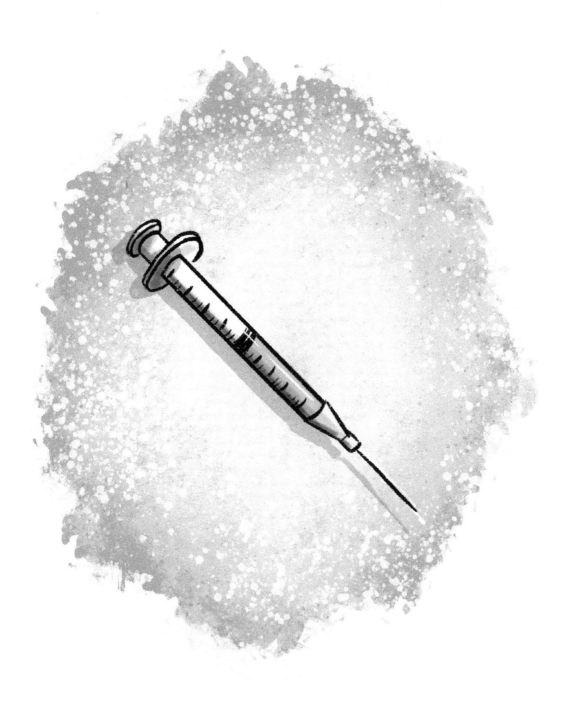

Still, I didn't want to roll up my sleeve.
I didn't want to get a shot.
I didn't want it to hurt.

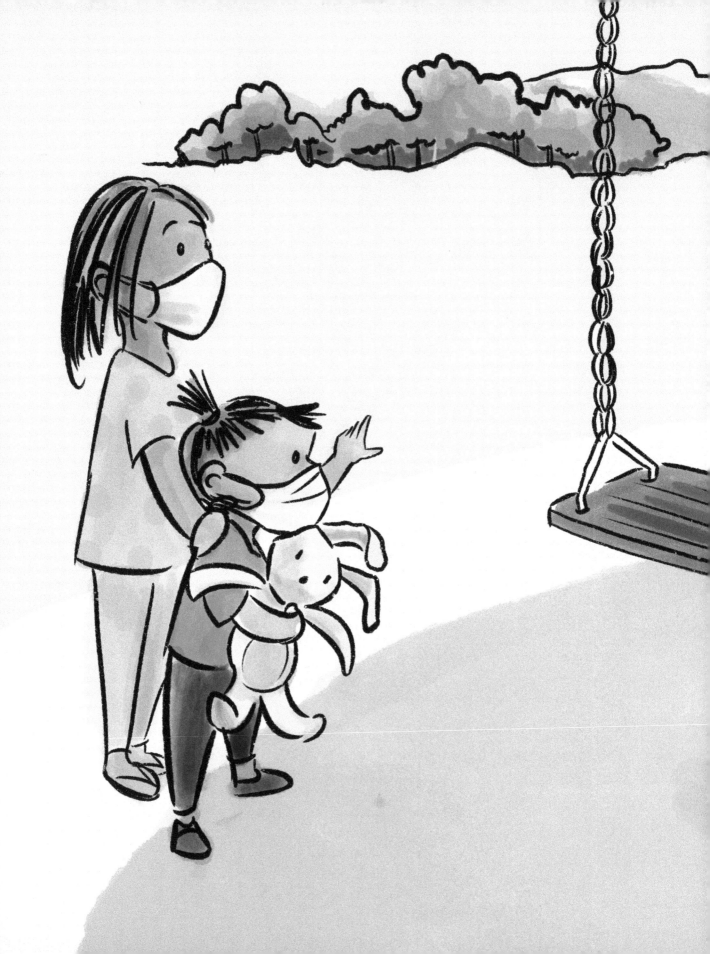

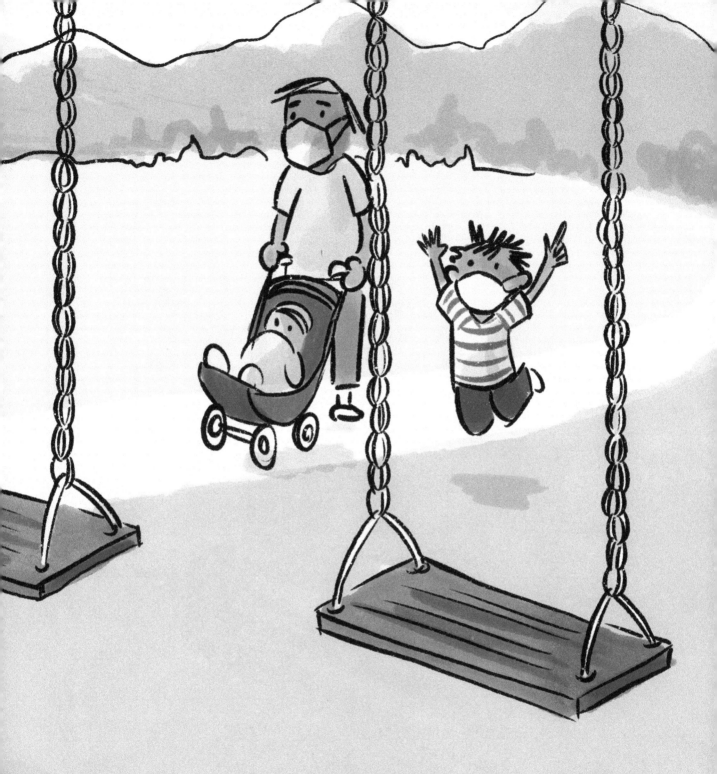

My friend, Wesley, wasn't allowed to get a Covid vaccine because of the way his body works.

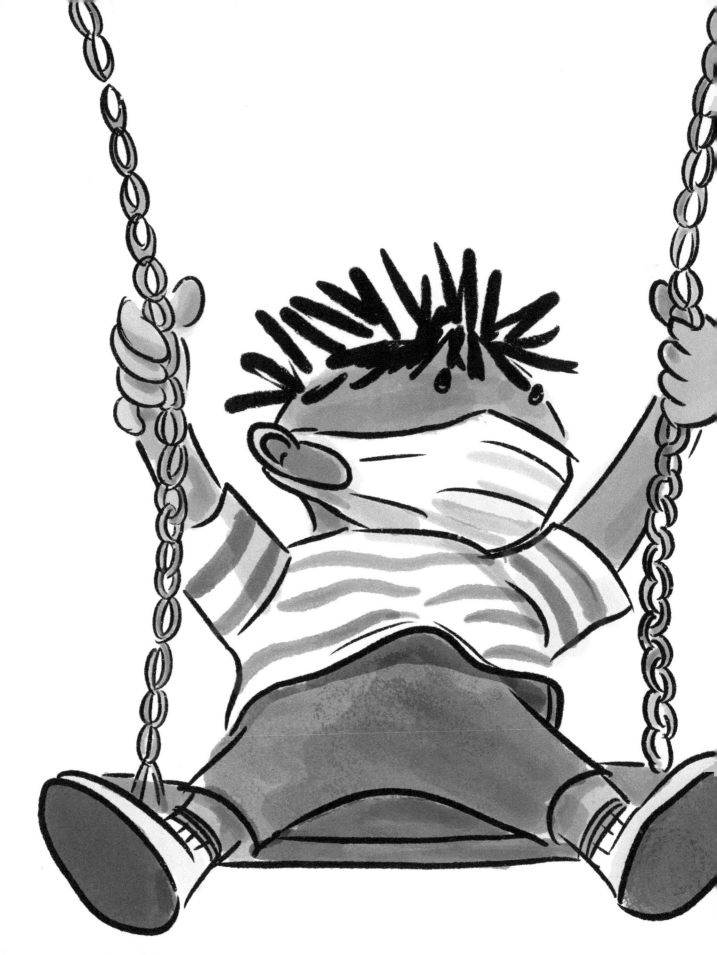

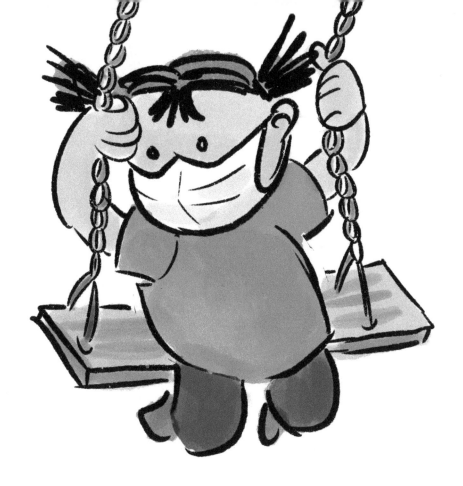

I told him he was lucky.

"You're the lucky one," said Wesley.
"You're healthy enough
for a vaccine. If I could get one,
I'd be the first one in line."

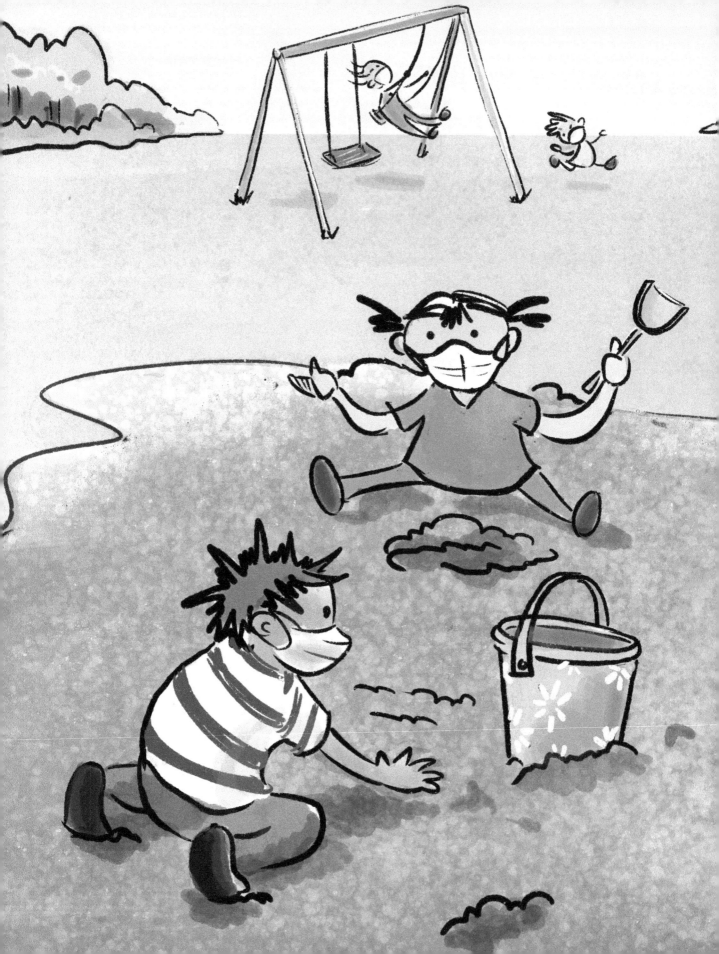

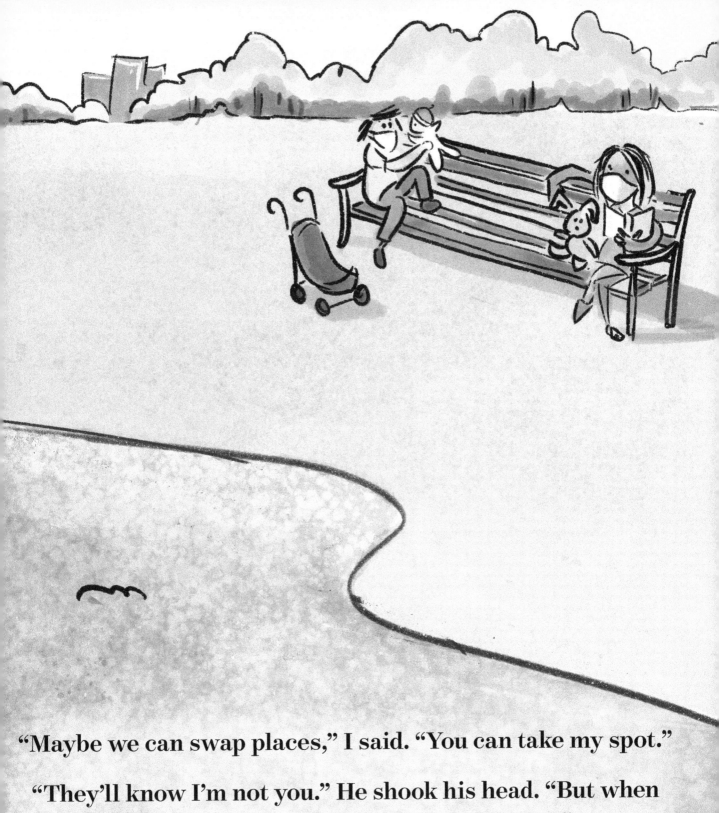

"Maybe we can swap places," I said. "You can take my spot."

"They'll know I'm not you." He shook his head. "But when you get your vaccine, it will help me, too."

"How does my shot help you?"

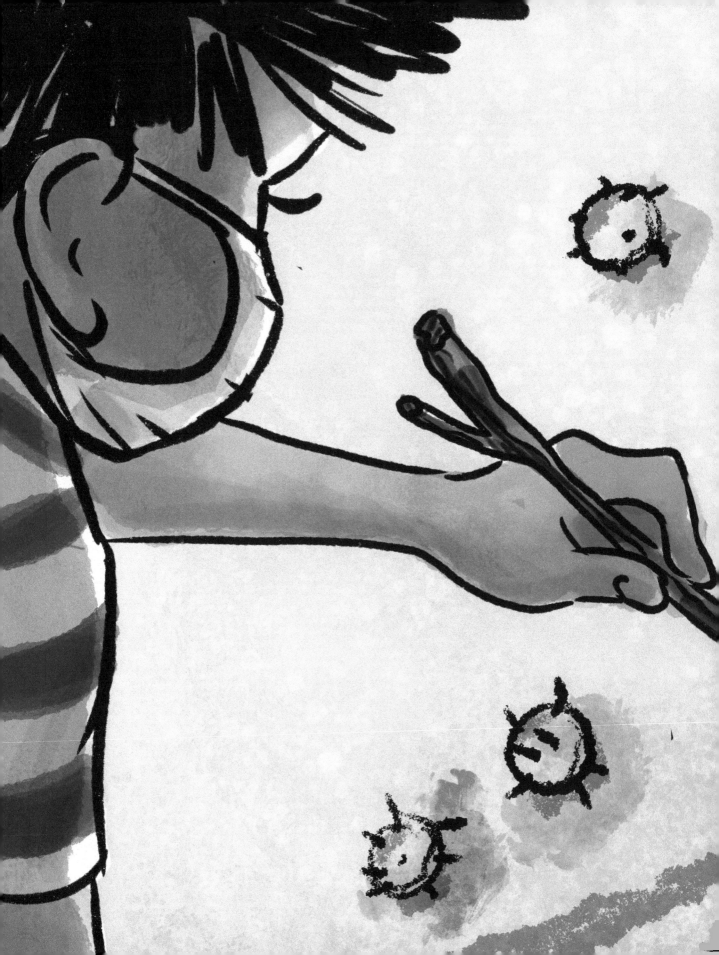

"A vaccine doesn't just stop Covid from spreading inside your body," he said. "It keeps the disease from spreading outside your body, too. With less germs floating in the air, I'm less likely to get sick."

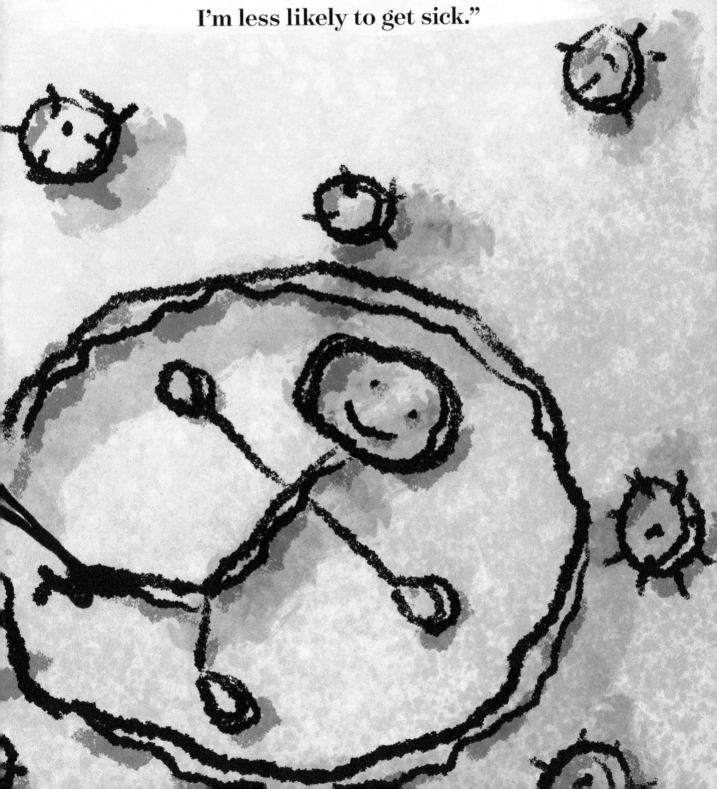

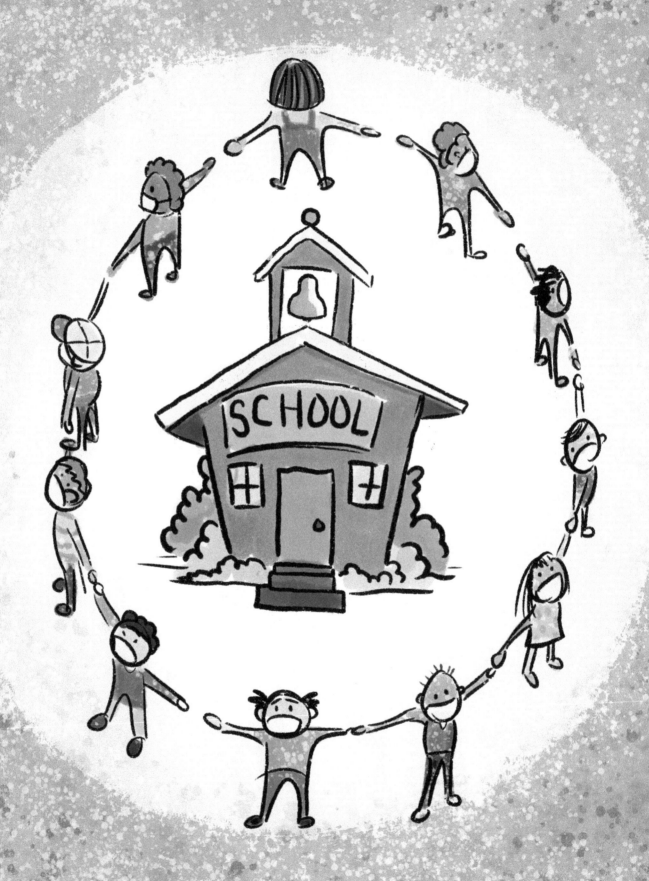

Wesley made a very good point.
His words got me thinking.

If enough people in our class
get vaccinated, it just might
protect the whole school.

If enough people in our neighborhood get vaccinated,
it just might protect the whole city.

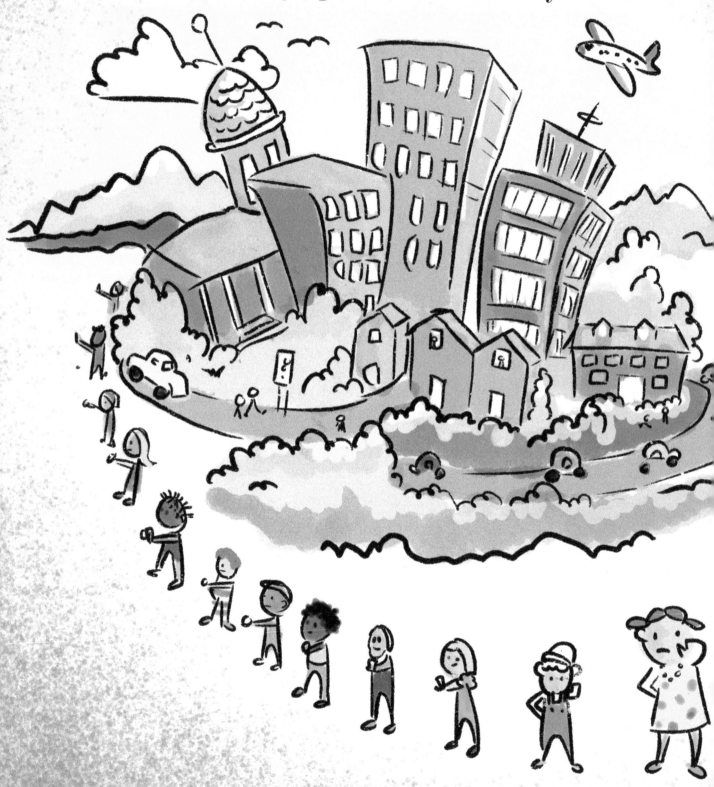

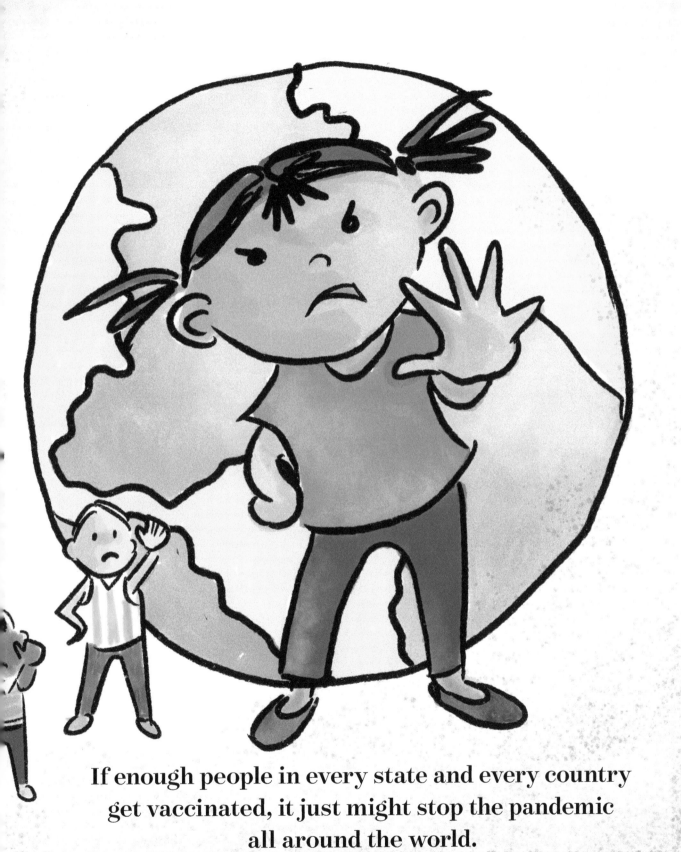

If enough people in every state and every country
get vaccinated, it just might stop the pandemic
all around the world.

So when it was time for my vaccine,

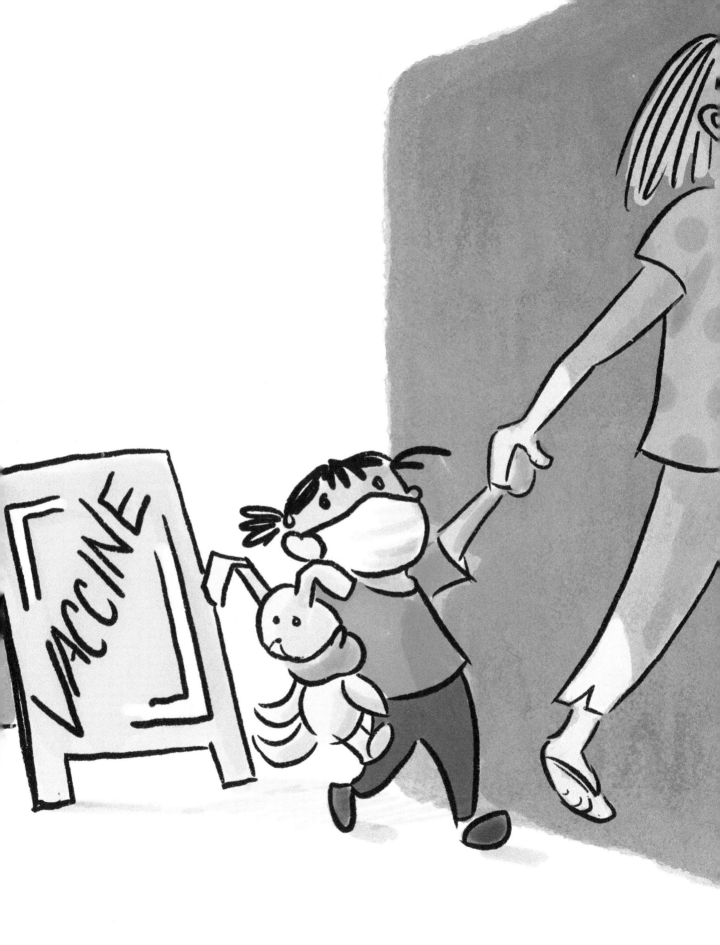

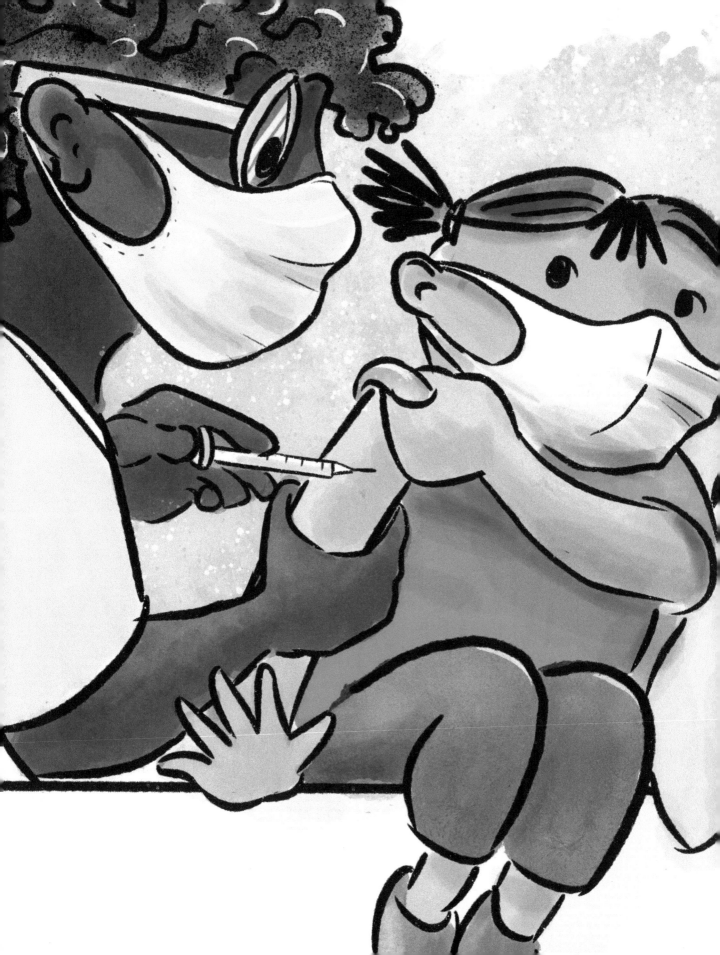

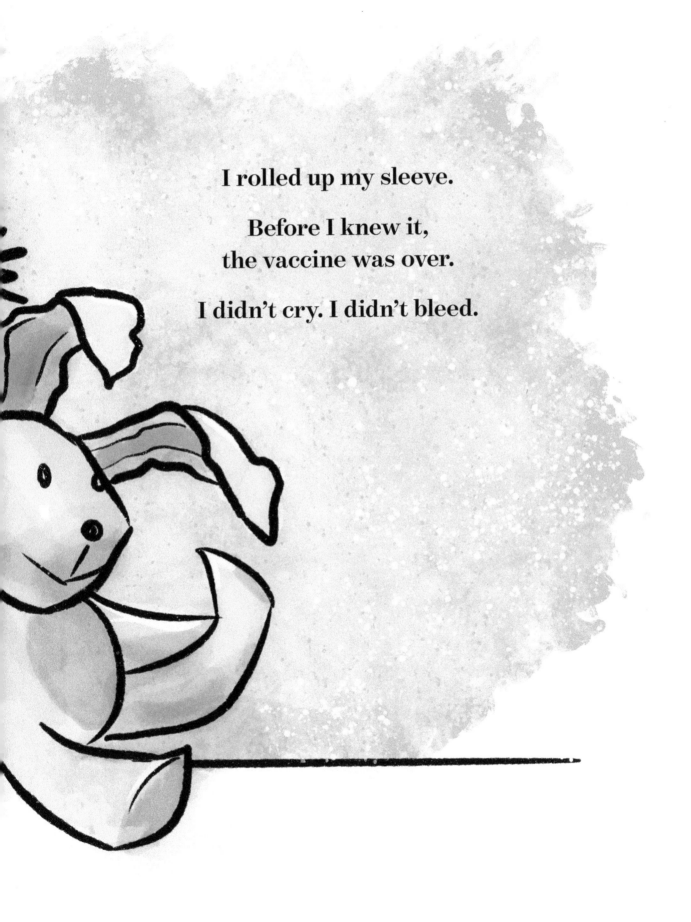

I rolled up my sleeve.

Before I knew it,
the vaccine was over.

I didn't cry. I didn't bleed.

It was just a tiny poke.

Of all the new things
I did during Covid,
this may have been the
tiniest of all.

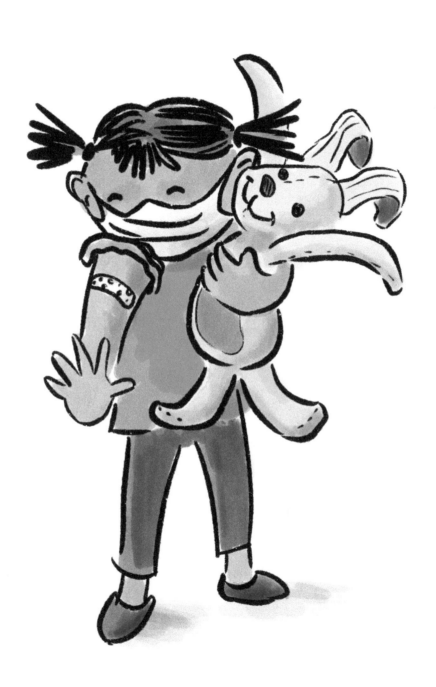

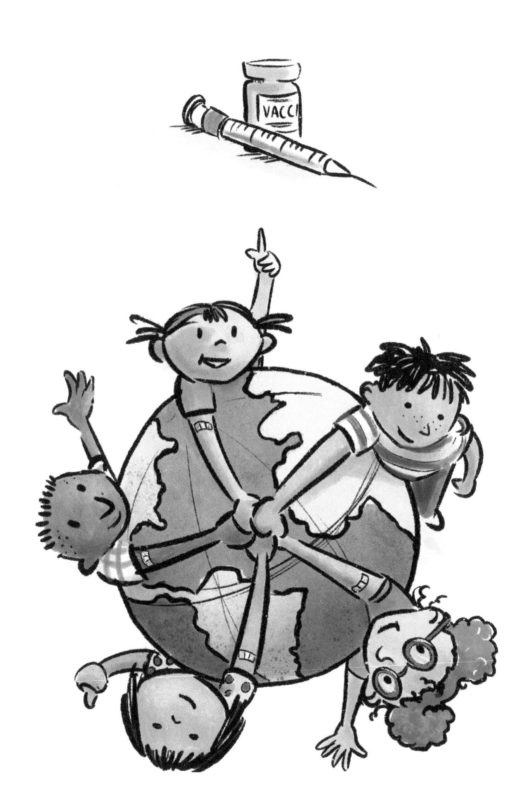

And if kids all over the globe
do this one tiny thing,
it can make a big difference
in helping the world get well.

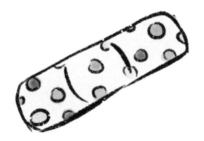

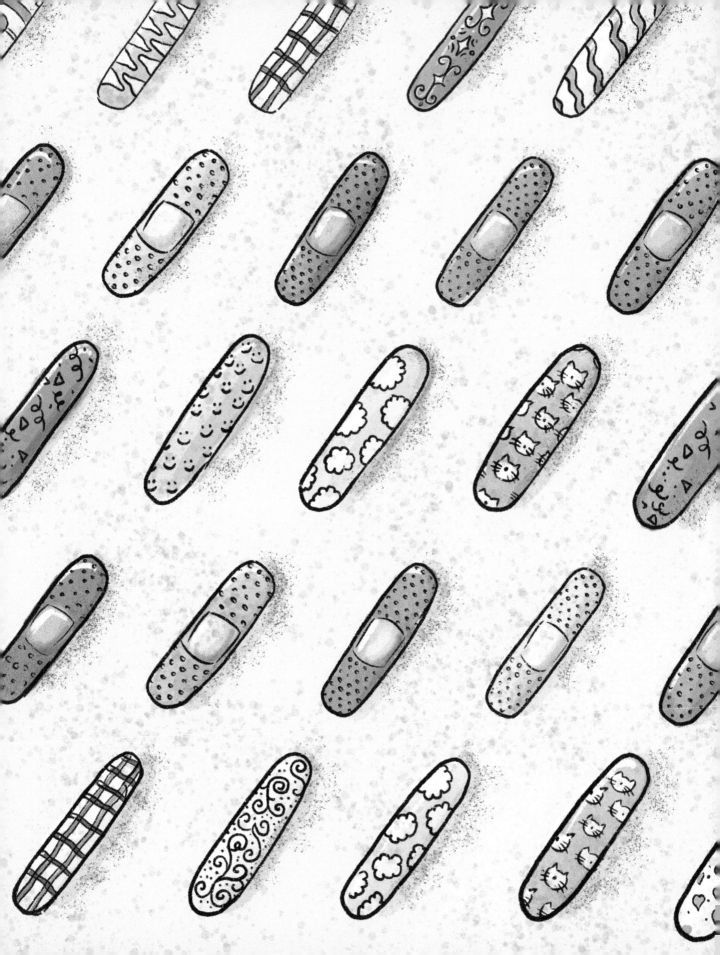

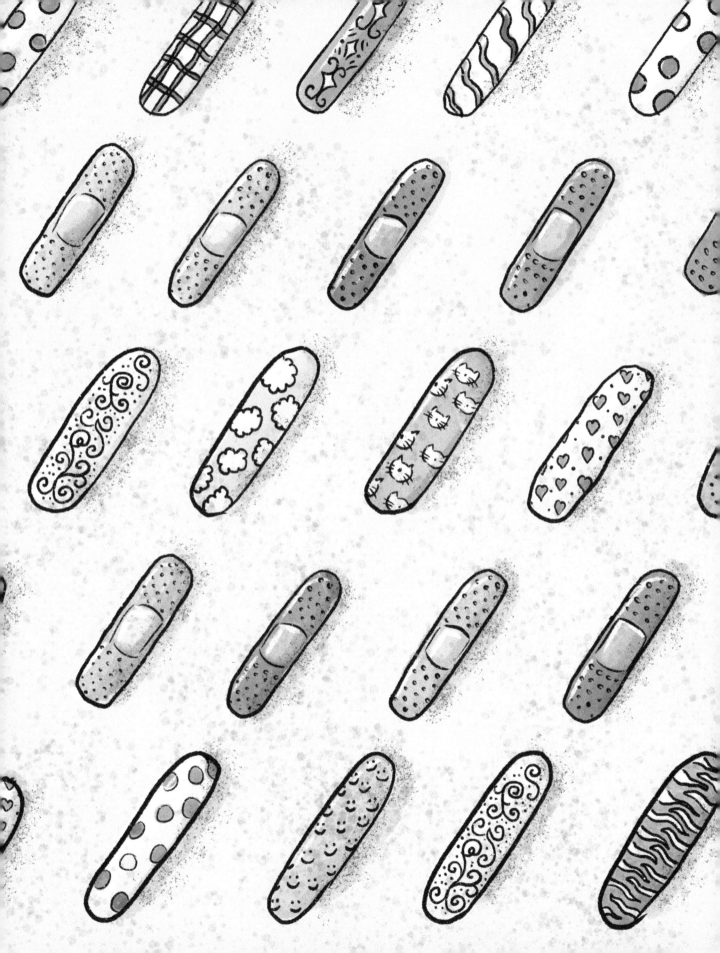

SOME FACTS ABOUT VACCINES

Vaccines protect people from getting sick by teaching our bodies to recognize and fight viruses. We call this protection *immunity*.

A vaccine doesn't just keep you from becoming sick. It also makes you unable to pass on the infection to other people.

Herd immunity occurs when enough people have had vaccines and the virus has no place to spread.

Herd immunity protects people who are unable to have a vaccine, people like Wesley in this story, or people whose immune systems don't work well, or people being treated with chemotherapy.

WHILE WE WAIT FOR HERD IMMUNITY, WE CAN SLOW THE SPREAD OF COVID-19

- Wear a mask when you go out.
- Stay six feet apart from people you don't live with.
- Wash your hands often with lots of soap and warm water.
- Do not attend large indoor gatherings.
- If you feel sick, stay home until you feel better or contact your doctor.

CPSIA information can be obtained
at www.ICGtesting.com
Printed in the USA
JSHW050523050921
18395JS00001B/1